Solutions for Erectile Dysfunction

Reducing or Eliminating Erectile Dysfunction in Older Men
by James Occhiogrosso, N.D., M.H.
North Fort Myers, Florida 33917
Author of "Your Prostate, Your Libido, Your Life"
Voice: 239-652-0421
Email: DrJim@HealthNaturallyToday.com
Website: http://www.HealthNaturallyToday.com[1]

I0426895

Solutions for Erectile Dysfunction

James Occhiogrosso

Published by James Occhiogrosso, 2018.

Also by James Occhiogrosso

Solutions for Erectile Dysfunction
Your Prostate, Your Libido, Your Life

Watch for more at www.prostatehealthnaturally.com/index.html.

Table of Contents

This book is dedicated to all my clients, many of whom patiently tested my thoughts and ideas to help with their own erectile dysfuntion issues

treated. The good news is that, in most cases, ED problems can be overcome with patience and perseverance. There are multiple natural substances, both nutritional and herbal, that can help to resolve the problem, but they must be taken at the correct dosage levels and for the correct issue. To have a good chance of rectifying ED, you must have a good handle on the cause.

Before getting into great detail, we might acknowledge that many ED symptoms can be quickly resolved with one of the FDA approved ED drugs. However, no drug actually cures the problem. At best, a drug covers up both symptoms and causes of the problem. Thus, over time, drugs allow the conditions that caused ED in the first place to become worse. Natural solutions can help the body heal by providing it with needed nutrients, and thus, can actually cure a problem.

I once gave a lecture about the potential long-term use of an ED drug allowing a circulatory problem to progress undetected for years. After the lecture, I was approached by a lady who told me her husband used increasing doses of an ED drug for many years. While the drug permitted a decent sex life, it also allowed his underlying cardiac problems to go unnoticed until a massive heart attack ended his life. In my opinion, the only way to use ED drugs—is as a crutch to get over the immediate issue—while you take steps to address underlying problems. Once the underlying problems are resolved, the ED drug is no longer needed.

PART I – ED Causes

Erectile dysfunction (ED) is generally defined as the inability of a
to attain or maintain an erection sufficient for vaginal penetration
satisfactory sexual performance. It is highly prevalent worldwide
affects most men in the age group of 30 thru 70 at some point in t
lives. ED is generally an age dependent issue effecting about 3-4%
men in their 30's and 40's to well over 50% of men over 65. This b
explores various issues that cause ED, presents some general soluti
and describes many nutritional elements, herbal supplements,
devices that can help a man with erectile dysfunction from any c
achieve a better sexual performance. Some of the information in
book comes from the chapters on ED from my book "Your Pros
Your Libido, Your Life", but there is considerable new informat
particularly that about devices and new medical treatments for Ere
Dysfunction based on research I've been doing and results from som
my clients.

By using this information presented here, a man with ED shoul
able to determine the approximate cause of his ED, and set a plan
resolving it.

It is unfortunate that unscrupulous supplement manufacturers
advantage of the suffering male with late night TV advertisement
worthless products—most of which contain one or two ingredients
research shows may have a positive effect on ED sufferers. The prob
with all of this is that the average male wants a quick fix, leaving
vulnerable to the manipulation of these advertisements
promise—but rarely deliver results—instant or otherwise. Yet, n
men fall victim to these advertisements promising an instant cure for
In my years of practice, the only instant action I've seen from any of tl
"quick fixes" — is how quickly they can take your money!

There are many external influences that affect ED. Thus, depenc
on the specific cause of your ED, there are also many ways it can

Determining an Approach to Solving ED

Any man with ED should first determine the most likely cause for his problem before attempting to rectify it. Using this approach, he can then determine the best path to try to rectify it. In general, there are five main causes of ED.

- **Natural Causes** — This can be a combination of aging, poor nutrition, lack of exercise, unrelated illnesses, circulatory issues and general poor health.
- **Medications** — Many prescription medications, especially anti-depressants and some cholesterol lowering drugs, as well as drugs for treating prostate conditions like BPH often can cause a loss of libido as well as ED.
- **Hormonal Imbalances** — a low free testosterone level coupled with a high estrogen level, can often cause a severe loss of sexual desire (libido) as well as problems getting and maintaining an erection. When ED is accompanied by a lack of vigor, poor muscle tone, depression, and low energy—all symptoms of declining testosterone levels—hormone testing and balancing is definitely in order.
- **Underlying Medical Conditions** — Many medical conditions can cause or exacerbate ED. Chief among these is uncontrolled diabetes, hypertension, or arteriosclerosis. Cardiac insufficiency is also a major cause. Its first symptom is often the onset of ED.
- **Medical Procedures or Physical Trauma** — Surgery for prostate, colon or rectal cancer, and any surgery in the pelvic area can disturb the nerves that are crucial for an erection. Even when surgery specifically tries to preserve nerve function, the ED can last a long time (sometimes years) or be totally irreversible. Spinal injuries as well as any physical trauma to the

3

pelvic area can also initiate ED. Depending on the amount of damage done, the condition may quickly resolve itself or be totally irreversible.

The first two items above can often be resolved with an improvement in nutrition and lifestyle, intelligent use of herbal preparations, and evaluation of prescription medications for side effects that cause ED. Often relatively minor changes can effect a major reversal of symptoms. This book also notes some medications known to have negative sexual side effects.

The third item, hormone balancing, requires testing of free hormone levels—especially testosterone, progesterone and estrogen—with a home saliva test kit. Such kits are available from my website and are quick and easy to use.

The last two items above represent illnesses or physical trauma, and are usually more difficult to overcome. However, in many cases trauma to the erectile nerves (medically known as neuropraxia) is not due to direct severing of the nerves, but simply that the nerves are in shock. In this case, there is much that can be done to accelerate the process of healing, often resulting in complete restoration of erectile function. See the sections on Vacuum Erection Devices, TENS therapy, Shock Wave therapy and Penile Implants below.

By categorizing your ED into one of the five broad groups detailed above, you can sub-categorize it further into one or more of the groups shown below. This may sound simple, but it is not. The causes of ED vary widely and you may need the help of your health professional to guide you. Once you have categorized the approximate (or exact) cause of your ED, you may be able to do the appropriate research, and by trial and error, resolve or at least improve your condition. Again, you may need the help of your health professional to guide you, but if you are doing it yourself, the information here should be of great help.

The causes of ED fall into some broadly defined categories. Working with your health practitioner, (a Naturopath, or Natural Health Practitioner if possible) you can approximate the root cause of your ED. Armed with that knowledge, you can then do your research to select nutrients and/or herbals supplements that might help with your condition. Note that all of the conditions listed overlap considerably.

Circulatory Issues

This is the most prevalent issue relating to lifestyle and general health, and is broadly defined as an issue of poor blood circulation. To achieve a satisfactory erection, a man must have relatively decent blood circulation throughout his body. The penis becomes erect through a series of neurological and physical processes. The neurological process occurs when the man becomes sexually aroused, which then triggers the physical process of inflating the penis with blood to achieve a sufficient erection. However, if arteries are clogged with plaque deposits they certainly cannot deliver adequate blood flow to the penis for an erection and thus, his erection is either weak, subsides quickly, or is non-existent. The most common circulatory issues that cause ED include but are not limited to the following conditions:

- High Blood Pressure, Diabetes, High Cholesterol, Lack of Exercise, Obesity, Smoking, excessive Alcohol use and Cardiac Insufficiency.

Any of these issues alone may cause ED, but in most cases, it is a combination of several of them that produce the problem. Of course, the above is a simplification of a very complex problem, but knowing that his ED may be caused by a seemingly unrelated problem goes a long way towards motivating a man to at least attempt to resolve the underlying problem.

Hormonal Imbalances

As a man ages, it is quite natural for him to encounter hormonal imbalances. This usually presents as a low free testosterone level, a high estrogen level or both. In any case, it is the ratio between testosterone and other hormones that typically causes a problem. Low testosterone levels usually cause a loss of libido in an aging man. Depending on how low his testosterone level is, it can also result in erectile dysfunction. The only way to know for sure is to have one's hormones tested. This can be done quite simply with a home saliva test kit. ED is often accompanied by a lack of vigor, poor muscle tone, depression, and low energy—all symptoms of declining testosterone levels.

Nutritional Deficiencies

This is one of the most difficult causes to pin down, but nutritional deficiencies, especially if severe, can directly cause ED. One of the most common is a zinc deficiency. While difficult to diagnose, nutritional deficiencies are the easiest to rectify. A blend of various vitamins and minerals as well as a few herbals may resolve the problem quite easily, albeit it may take a few months for the improved nutrition to make an effect.

Pharmaceutical Medications

Many medications, particularly those used for prostate problems, as well as anti-depressants and some statin drugs can directly cause a loss of libido or ED. If you are taking any prescription medications, it is prudent for you to research each one for its effects on sexual performance. Many men simply ask their doctors about this and almost always get a negative or non-definitive answer. Doctors are often in denial about the side effects of the medications they prescribe and drug representatives rarely give their doctor clients a clear picture of them, whether they know about them or not. The only solution is to do the research yourself, or visit a health practitioner that is well aware of medication side effects or will research them for you.

Surgery or Trauma

Treatment for prostate or other cancer that involves surgery or radiation is well known to be a cause of ED subsequent to or concurrent with the treatment. To resolve such ED requires a high degree of motivation as well as a good working knowledge of the physiology of an erection and possibly the cooperation of your doctor. There are many different techniques for restoring function lost thru surgery or radiation.

Emotional Issues

A man may experience ED as a result of emotional problems, particularly stress. Often, a man will suffer temporary erectile dysfunction due to the stress of a divorce, loss of a job, death of a loved one, or simply the stress of living. In cases like this, the ED usually vanishes when the stress issue causing it is resolved. If an anti-depressant is prescribed, research it so you can take the lowest dose that will help you, without exacerbating your ED problem. If the drug causes deterioration in performance, tell your doctor immediately, so it can be changed to one that doesn't affect you as much.

Summary of Part One

Erectile Dysfunction is a serious problem that has a profound emotional effect on both the suffering man and his significant other. In many cases, a man's doctor is not very sensitive to his suffering, and if a prescription drug doesn't help, his arsenal for fixing the problem is essentially empty.

Fortunately, there are many natural substances as well as medical devices and treatments that can help a man suffering from ED. Unfortunately, it may take a course of trial and error to determine what works and what doesn't, or to find a doctor willing to work with you.

Part Two of this book provides more detailed information on nutritional items and herbal supplements known to help with ED, as well as FDA approved drugs and other medical solutions like Vacuum Erection Devices, Penile Implants, TENS and Shock Wave Therapy.

Some of these approaches show promise and there may be clinical studies starting soon in the U.S. The Shock Wave therapy described in Part Two, in particular shows much promise and is approved in Canada.

A motivated guy suffering from Erectile Dysfunction (ED) will find a multitude of ways to try to resolve his problem in Part 2 of this book, and, hopefully, find one that will work for him.

PART II – Fighting ED

Part Two of this book provides a guy suffering from Erectile Dysfunction (ED) a multitude of ways to try to resolve his problem. It discusses in detail nutritional items and herbal supplements that are known to help, as well as FDA drugs and medical devices that one can investigate if the natural approaches fail.

Some of the information in this article is condensed information from my book "Your Prostate, Your Libido, Your Life". Other information, particularly that about devices and new medical treatments for Erectile Dysfunction is based on new research I've been doing and results from some of my clients.

Unfortunately, due to the widespread nature of this problem, advertising for products that are of dubious benefit persuades many men to try them wasting both their time and money. But, since there is lots of money to be made—such products certainly dominate the market.

Many guys, on first encountering ED, will either rush to their nearest health food store and load up on a bunch of (often useless) male enhancement supplements, make an appointment with the doctor to have their testosterone level checked, or push their doctor for a prescription for an ED drug. While this may resolve the immediate problem, it is rarely a long-term solution.

The goal of this book is to help you determine the approximate cause of your ED, (in Part 1) and then, armed with that information, apply this knowledge in an intelligent way to help rectify your ED.

About ED

Erectile dysfunction (ED), also known as impotence, is generally defined as the inability of a man to attain or maintain an erection sufficient for vaginal penetration and satisfactory sexual performance. It is highly prevalent worldwide and affects a high percentage of aging men. This book describes many solutions for ED, both natural and medical, targeted toward correcting a specific underlying cause. It assumes you have researched the cause(s) of your ED problem either by yourself, or with the help of your health provider, and that you have a handle on the most likely cause of your ED. It discusses nutritional supplements, herbal remedies, ED drugs, and mechanical devices that can help minimize or resolve problems associated with ED.

In addition to nutritional or herbal items, many men have had good success using pelvic floor exercises (also known as Kegel exercises) to help overcome erectile dysfunction. It is beyond the scope of this article explain these exercises, but an excellent discussion of them can be found in *The Testosterone Syndrome* by Eugene Shippen, M.D.

Risk factors for age-related ED are generally the same as those for cardiac issues. In fact, ED can be considered to be a precursor to heart problems. A man with ED may be able to improve his sexual performance using natural products. This includes dietary changes, and the addition of vitamins and herbal supplements. Unfortunately, the list of items that *"may be helpful"* is long, and few men take the time to experiment and determine what works for them and what doesn't.

This rush towards a quick fix for their ED often makes men vulnerable to claims made for supplements and herbal remedies advertised in late-night TV commercials for correcting ED. The vast majority of these claims are false or misleading, and in general, most of the products are worthless.

However, this is not to say that all nutritional supplements and herbal remedies are useless. Many of them have solid science to establish their efficacy, and many of them are very helpful for problems like ED, especially when the source is a nutritional deficiency.

Unfortunately, many unscrupulous supplement suppliers take advantage of weak science to write extremely positive and misleading advertising for products that do very little. I recently noticed a very persuasive advertisement about a product named Cyvita, touted as a cure-all for ED. The product primarily contains—as its active ingredient—L-Carnitine (or Carnitine) a common natural amino acid. While Carnitine can be useful as part of a complete nutritional rehabilitation program aimed at resolving ED, I have never seen any evidence that used alone—it will have a noticeable effect on ED. However, an advertisement can say almost anything, as long as they stay within certain bounds of truth, but there is a huge disconnect between a fact and a misleading statement. Stating that Carnitine might help ED is true, but spinning weak science into virtual cure, is, to say the least, quite misleading.

It is imperative that the reader first knows the approximate source of his ED before attempting to rectify it. Men often jump into ordering products that may be quite effective for one cause of ED, but useless for another. If, for example, low levels of nitric oxide are causing your erectile dysfunction, the amino acids arginine or citrulline may help. On the other hand, if your problem is low libido due to low testosterone levels, then supplemental amino acids will be of little value. Without a decent guess at the source of your ED, you may spend considerable money and waste a lot of time trying products that have little chance of helping. If you decide to use natural substances, keep in mind they tend to work slowly, and may not work the same in all individuals.

The balance of this book explores solutions for the problem of Erectile Dysfunction. It discusses many nutritional supplements, herbal remedies, drugs, and some mechanical devices that may help you reduce or even eliminate the problem. Before using the information in this book to attempt to rectify your ED, you should have a good handle on the source of your ED from Part One. If you don't, I strongly suggest you go back and read Part One again. If you do not know what the cause of your ED is, you will likely waste a lot of time, money and effort with little chance of resolving it.

Health Conditions, Lifestyle and Hormones

Most men have few problems with erectile dysfunction in their youth and expect such youthful vigor to continue forever. However, as the years advance, the health and vitality of the body deteriorates, and the level of sexual vigor drops accordingly. Unfortunately, many men suffering from erectile dysfunction or loss of libido, cannot (or will not) admit to a connection between their overall health and their sexual problems. Fortunately, most such problems can be corrected. [1]

Many cases of erectile dysfunction are due to impaired blood circulation resulting from an underlying health condition. All body organs and tissues depend on circulating blood to provide necessary nutrients and remove waste products. An organ lacking good blood circulation cannot maintain peak health. The overall health of the bodies circulation system is critical for satisfactory sexual performance.

Disruption of hormone levels, particularly when testosterone levels are low, can result in poor sexual function and loss of libido. However, while low testosterone levels can affect erectile performance, more often the problem is a side effect of other health conditions. Impotence (erectile dysfunction) is often caused by seemingly unrelated health conditions or is a side effect of medical treatment. Many medications, especially antidepressants, can cause or exacerbate it. Thus, an unwary man can easily become trapped in a vicious cycle. Low testosterone levels can cause depression as well as a decrease in libido. If his depression is treated with antidepressants, his libido may decrease even more, and he may experience medication-related erectile dysfunction, further increasing his depression and compounding his problems. [2] [3] [4] [5] [6] [7]

An erection is wholly dependent on good blood circulation. The penis requires unimpeded blood circulation to produce an erection for sexual activity. Thus, while some cases of erectile dysfunction are related to low testosterone, more often it is a direct result of poor health and impaired blood circulation. Any health condition, medication, or physical injury that impedes blood circulation in a man can result in erectile dysfunction. Erectile dysfunction is often the first symptom of a compromised vascular system, and can be an early symptom of cardiovascular problems. [8]

Several studies have found erectile dysfunction to be prevalent among men with high total cholesterol and low HDL/LDL ratios. High cholesterol and triglyceride levels are well known as strong risk factors for numerous cardiovascular problems. Reducing their levels can help correct erectile dysfunction while also lowering the risk of other problems. Often, high cholesterol and trigliceride levels are accompanied by or result in high blood pressure (hypertension), hardening of the arteries (arteriosclerosis), or arteries clogged by cholesterol deposits (atherosclerosis). These conditions all inhibit blood flow in the body and the penis, and are grouped under the general term of vascular or cardiovascular dysfunction.

Diabetes can also cause serious problems. It exacerbates erectile dysfunction by making blood vessels less elastic, and less able to dilate fully, thus restricting blood flow during an erection. It also deteriorates nerve viability, decreasing the sensitivity of the penis and often creating problems with achieving orgasm. Both effects are magnified when the condition has been present or poorly controlled for many years. Diabetes also has profound effects on the endocrine system, and thus, on hormone levels. Studies have shown men with ED have lowered levels of the pituitary hormones that control testosterone production, and thus, lower levels of free testosterone. Long-term uncontrolled diabetes nearly always leads to ED.

Sarcopenia is a normal aspect of aging and is defined as a gradual decrease in the ability to maintain muscle function and mass. It is generally an age-related deterioration, but certain conditions like congestive heart failure, certain liver conditions, and hormone deficiencies, particularly of testosterone in a man, can cause or accelerate it. While it is not actually a disease, it is a predisposing factor for injuries in the elderly as well as sexual performance and quality of life issues. Good health via proper nutrition and exercise as well as maintaining proper levels of testosterone and other hormones can help delay or minimize it.

Similarly, the blockage of veins and arteries due to arteriosclerosis and atherosclerosis can cause or exacerbate impotence by physically diminishing blood flow to the penis. Hypertension is frequently the result of clogged arteries from either condition. When the body's circulation system is clogged with deposits, the heart must pump harder to move blood around the body, thus raising blood pressure. And even though the heart is pumping harder, blood flow is still diminished from normal. It is my firm belief that erectile dysfunction is a precursor to more serious problems, and that correcting it can and should be done naturally, with minimum use of drugs.

Critical Nutritional Items

It is evident from research that ED is caused by a combination of factors; some nutritional, some lifestyle, and some as side effects of other clinical conditions. In addition, there is much overlap between items that are typically called lifestyle factors and those that are deemed nutritional. For example, eating habits can be considered to span both the lifestyle and nutritional category.

A man whose ED appears to be from some kind of nutritional deficiency or a blood circulation problem may be helped by a combination of vitamins, herbs, minerals and other nutrients that will support the bodies natural systems.

There are many critical nutrients that are essential for good health as well as good sexual function. To list them all here would require many more pages than this article is allotted. However, most of them can be obtained from a high quality multi-vitamin/multi-mineral like our Life Essentials product. This includes many products sold in quality health food stores, and excludes many multi-vitamin products sold in drug store and supermarket chains.

A good multi-vitamin/multi-mineral product will generally cost about $50 for a two-month supply. A general rule for determining quality is to look at the ingredients part of its label. High quality products list the source of most of their vitamins and minerals, and usually have few additives. For example; Vitamin E is actually a group of 8 fractions. Typically, multi-vitamin products only provide one of them—alpha-tocopherol. With inexpensive vitamin products, the source is not listed or is DL-alpha-tocopherol, a synthetic analog. Quality multi-vitamin products will use D-alpha-tocopherol, the natural form, which has been established to be more than two-three times more absorbable by the human body than the synthetic analog. Also, quality multi-vitamin products provide small dosages of many trace minerals, do not use fillers, and rarely use artificial coloring.

Unfortunately, it is a formidable (and often impossible) task to determine nutrient deficiencies that cause ED with absolute certainty. A few specific nutrient deficiencies (like Zinc) have been positively linked to ED, and there is much evidence linking it to hormone imbalances, especially testosterone deficiency. What remains unknown is all of the mechanisms that cause such imbalances. Some are obvious while others are subtle.

When it comes to erectile dysfunction, many men fall into "one size fits all" thinking. The paradigm in the U.S. and other western countries is that a single solution or pill can fix everything. Nothing could be further from the truth. ED is a multifactorial problem that can be based on nutritional deficiencies, illness and/or many other bodily disturbances. If you are suffering from ED, the first step for a natural solution is to start supplementing with quality vitamins and minerals to overcome any nutritional deficiencies. A natural health practitioner can help you determine where any deficiencies may be hiding.

There are many vitamins and minerals that are necessary for the maintenance of life. Some of these are micronutrients where the body needs a very small amount, while others are macronutrients where much larger quantities are needed. Supplements of micronutrients are typically measured in micrograms (mcg) and macronutrients in milligrams (mg.). It is impossible to discuss all of the vitamins, minerals and other nutrients vital to human health without writing many thousands of pages.

The best way to get most of the micronutrients needed for supplementation is to purchase a quality multi-vitamin product. One important criterion in selecting a multivitamin is to be aware that a day's supply of many needed macronutrients (like calcium) often cannot fit into a small capsule. Thus, many "one-a-day" type vitamin tablets are limited in value. Most quality multivitamins require three to six capsules per day to reach optimal nutrient quantities. It is also important to understand that vitamin supplements are just—supplements, and they don't provide therapeutic doses of anything.

You cannot expect to maintain good health by taking vitamins and eating poorly. Vitamin and other food supplements are not substitutes for good dietary and lifestyle habits and an adequate intake of vitamins, minerals, and other nutrients from food and supplements is essential for good health as well as erectile function. Supplementing a multivitamin-multimineral product with some specific nutrients to help ED can be very rewarding. Below is a list of items that have good science regarding their efficacy. The items are not listed in any particular order and all are critical for good health.

Specific Vitamins for ED.

Vitamins B and C

Deficiencies in any of these vitamins can contribute to ED. Most people do not consume an optimal amount of these vitamins through their diet alone. Elderly or chronically ill adults or those with malabsorption problems are at increased risk of severe deficiencies, particularly of B vitamins. The B-vitamin family is noted for enhancing nerve communication. With ED, nerve communication can be suppressed, and B-vitamins can sometimes help.

Vitamin C is a strong antioxidants. Deficiencies are associated with poor circulation and heart disease and can increase the risk of erectile dysfunction. Vitamin E, in particular is known to help thin the blood, allowing for better blood circulation. Since poor circulation is often a contributing cause for ED, it is prudent to make sure your vitamin E levels are adequate.

Erectile dysfunction is often the first symptom of a cardiovascular problem, and may appear long before the latter is diagnosed. Thus, any improvement in the ability of blood vessels to dilate or any lowering of blood pressure can be a major step toward restoring general health—as well as reducing ED. This is particularly evident in those who smoke. Nicotine constricts blood vessels and produces free radicals that rapidly use up vitamin C. Thus, smokers are at increased risk for vitamin C deficiency.

There is much evidence that vitamin C has significant value for treating vascular problems. A daily intake of 500 mg of vitamin C (several times the RDA) can improve blood vessel dilation. The ability of blood vessels to dilate is crucial to proper sexual performance and is a strong contributing factor for ED. Studies also show that vitamin C can lower blood pressure and help reduce problems with coronary artery disease

Vitamin E

This is actually a family of related compounds, four tocopherols and four tocotrienols. Recent research on the effects of the tocotrienol fractions strongly indicates they can help with many other problems. One study found that tocotrienols could help clear blockages in the carotid arteries (the main suppliers of blood to the brain), potentially reducing the risk of stroke. [9] Others have shown that tocotrienols can reduce the level of low-density lipoproteins (LDL), the bad form of cholesterol in the blood, as well as improve nervous system communication. [10][11] Narrowing of arteries in the human body do not occur in isolation. If there are deposits in the carotid arteries, then it is likely that similar problems exist in penile arteries. Thus, tocotrienols may help with erectile dysfunction caused by impaired blood circulation and clogged arteries. It is important to take only natural vitamin E supplements, prefixed with "d" instead of "dl." Most over-the-counter vitamin E products, especially inexpensive ones, contain only synthetic alpha-tocopherol (dl-alpha-tocopherol). Thus, the benefits derived from taking them are, at best, marginal. Acceptable vitamin E supplements contain at least the four tocopherol components of natural vitamin E. Better supplements also have all four tocotrienol fractions derived from palm oil.

Unfortunately, the RDA for most vitamins and minerals continues to be based on the prevention of deficiency diseases, rather than on enhancing health or prevention of chronic illness. Most experts agree that the RDAs are far too low for the prevention of chronic diseases, though there is disagreement on what the optimum levels of various nutrients are. Many natural health professionals recommend increased intake of nutrients far in excess of their RDA, especially when the body is abnormally stressed. In most cases, such levels are safe.

To maintain good health, natural health professionals recommend a quality multi-vitamin/multi-mineral product, along with a B-Complex product containing approximately 100 mg of the essential B vitamins,

2000-3000 mg of vitamin C, and a Vitamin E complex that contains all 8 fractions of vitamin E with 800 IU of D-Alpha-tocopherol.

Vitamin D

This vitamin controls many interrelated body processes, and has profound effects on the immune system. Many researchers suggest it should be called a hormone and several books have called it the "sunshine hormone."

The primary way the human body gets vitamin D is from the sun. Human beings have a built in mechanism for obtaining vitamin D through the action of sunlight on their exposed skin. Insufficient sun exposure results in vitamin D deficiency. Many experts estimate that more than 80 percent of the U.S. population is severely deficient in vitamin D, especially during the winter months.

In many studies, vitamin D supplementation has been shown to improve the outcome for people with cardiovascular problems, arthritis, depression, diabetes, hypertension, kidney problems, cancer, and other chronic conditions. [12] [13] [14] [15] [16] [17]

Few foods contain significant amounts of vitamin D, and unfortunately, those that do are typically not consumed in sufficient quantity by much of the population. Thus, obtaining sufficient vitamin D solely from food is difficult, if not impossible, particularly in light of the nutrient-poor fast foods many people consume. In addition, aging contributes to deficiencies in older individuals by reducing the body's ability to synthesize vitamin D from sunlight. [18]

During winter months in the U.S., it is virtually impossible to get sufficient sunlight to forestall a vitamin D deficiency, even for those with fair skin. The only real exception to this is for folks that live in southern Florida, southern Texas, or Hawaii. Nearly everyone living north of these areas is subject to a vitamin D deficiency for the greater part of the year.

People who live in northern areas can supplement during the winter months, or when they cannot get out into the sun regularly. Most over-the-counter multivitamins sold today contain 200 to 400

International Units (IU) of Vitamin D. According to the latest research, this is insufficient. Most experts recommend 1000 to 2000 IU daily and many recommend more. the safe upper limit for vitamin D is currently acknowledged to be about 10,000.

Essential Fatty Acids

There are many essential fatty acids (EFAs), called "essential" because the human body does not manufacture them and thus it is essential that they come from the diet. Omega-3 and omega-6 are, by far, the most critical and typically the ones subject to serious imbalances. The human body works best on a diet that has about a 1:1 ratio of omega-3 to omega-6. Unfortunately, highly processed foods tend to skew this ratio. As a result, most Westerners get far too much omega-6, and far too little omega-3 in their diets. [19]

Meat consumption (particularly processed meats) and many other highly processed dietary items cause the ratio of omega-6 to omega-3 to become skewed. Vegetable oils produced from corn, soy, safflower, and sunflower—the predominant oils in use today—are composed mostly of omega-6.

Some good plant sources of omega-3 are: (in order of highest omega-3 content): flax seed, extra virgin olive oil, coconut oil, and avocados. Organic butter or cheese made from the milk of grass-fed cows is also a good source. The best animal sources are cold-water fish like salmon.

Omega-3 fatty acids are also abundant in most nuts and seeds, and in dark green leafy vegetables. Many of the food and herbal items that help with chronic diseases have high levels of omega-3. Omega-6 deficiencies are rare and supplementation is not typically required. The human body works best when everything is in balance. Just like hormone ratios, it is the balance between omega-6 and omega-3 that is critical. Both are essential and necessary for life.

Amino Acids

L-Arginine (or arginine) — is a semi-essential amino acids prevalent in virtually all protein-rich foods, particularly nuts, seeds, fish, and beans. Arginine, being semi-essential, can be made by the body but is also an important element in the diet especially for men with ED. Arginine acts as an agent to help increase nitric oxide (NO) levels in the blood.

Normally, nitric oxide is abundant in the body, but aging or poor diet can result in inadequate production.[20] Without sufficient nitric oxide levels, it is impossible for a man to have and sustain an erection. Men with decreased levels of nitric oxide almost always suffer from erectile dysfunction. [21][22][23][24][25]

Nitric oxide acts to relax and dilate the smooth muscle tissue of penile arteries thus allowing sufficient blood flow into the penis for an erection. By helping increase the body's levels of nitric oxide, arginine can often resolve problems with erectile dysfunction. Studies have shown that about three to six grams of arginine daily can help restore erectile function for most men.[26]

L-Citrulline or Citrulline — Citrulline is another amino acid that is an integral part of nitric oxide synthesis and strongly related to arginine. In many tissues of the body that produce nitric oxide, citrulline is converted to arginine. Thus, supplemental citrulline can increase the availability of arginine. Oral supplementation with citrulline, as an amino acid precursor to arginine, can raise blood levels of arginine, and subsequently increase total available nitric oxide, greatly enhancing the potential for a normal erection in a man with erectile dysfunction. In addition, supplementation with both arginine and citrulline can help reduce many age-related problems with circulation.

Both Arginine and Citrulline can help increase blood circulation through arteries clogged with cholesterol. This is an important consideration for ED, as well as for men with cardiac insufficiencies. Studies have found supplemental arginine and citrulline helpful for reducing age-related heart damage, cholesterol levels, and systolic blood pressure in both animals and humans.

> *Caution*: *Arginine and Carnitine should not be used in conjunction with ED drugs or by someone being treated for a heart condition without consulting a health professional first.*

L-Carnitine or Carnitine — This amino acid is typically associated with muscle building and an increase in exercise tolerance. However, studies have shown that it has a positive effect on nocturnal penile tumescence, erectile function, and libido.

Note: Amino acids should be taken in relatively high doses and for at least 1-2 months before any effect would be noticed. Follow directions on the bottle. Arginine is typically 3-5 gms per day, while Citrulline and Carnitine are usually about 1-2 gms/day

Critical Minerals

Selenium — An important dietary trace element, selenium has been found to be protective against both breast and prostate disease. A healthy prostate is essential for good erectile function.

A recent study examined the relationship between selenium and the alpha and gamma tocopherol fractions of vitamin E. Blood samples from 117 men that developed prostate cancer were compared to samples from a control group of 233 men. The study found a protective effect with the alpha-tocopherol fraction of vitamin E. However, of greater significance was the finding that men with the highest levels of gamma-tocopherol had a five-to-one reduction in the risk for developing prostate cancer as compared to those with the lowest levels. Also noted was that the statistically significant protection offered by high levels of selenium and alpha-tocopherol occurred only when gamma-tocopherol levels were also high. [27] Synergy between various vitamin E fractions and selenium has been noted in other studies as well.

The recommended daily intake of selenium is 55 mcg, with an upper safe limit of 400 mcg. Many experts recommend between 100 and 200 micrograms (mcg) per day though the significant protective effect appears to be at the higher intake level.

Zinc — is an essential trace element that plays an important role in many body processes. Studies have found that men with prostate disease have lower levels of zinc in their bodies than healthy men. According to Michael Murray, N.D., the author of Male Sexual Vitality—*Chronic prostate infections are often linked to a lack of dietary zinc.* Prostate glands containing cancer generally have lower levels of zinc than healthy glands.

There are many processes in the body involved in the repair of DNA that require zinc to function properly. It is an important regulator of many metabolic processes in the body. Studies have found that low testosterone levels generally accompany low levels of zinc in the prostate. [28]

Most foods contain small amounts of zinc. Processed foods lose most of their zinc in the processing. Legumes, seeds, and nuts contain relatively high amounts of zinc and selenium and are worthwhile additions to your diet. Pumpkin seeds in particular are a good source of zinc. The daily recommended dietary allowance (RDA) of zinc for men is 12 to 15 milligrams. But many experts recommend higher levels in the order of 25 to 80 mg/day for optimum health. As with most nutrients, older adults need more zinc than younger ones. [29] Unfortunately, there is considerable disagreement over what the ODA for zinc should be. Until this is defined better, it is prudent to keep your total daily intake of zinc to around 50 mg per day.

About Testosterone

A popular misconception of many men is that low testosterone causes all erectile dysfunction. ED is caused by multiple factors, many of which have nothing to do with testosterone levels. However, since it is one of the causes, and it is relatively easy to test hormone levels with a home saliva test kit, it is prudent to start with a hormone test. If your levels are in the normal range, your ED is most likely coming from other sources. Specifically, low free testosterone coupled with high estrogen, can often cause a severe loss of sexual desire (libido) as well as problems getting and maintaining an erection.

Testosterone is an extremely important hormone for the overall health of the human body and is particularly critical for male sexual ability and satisfaction. A recent large study noted an increase in general overall mortality of about fifteen percent for men with low testosterone levels as compared to men with normal levels. [30] Common symptoms of low free testosterone are an inability (or reduced ability) to have an orgasm during normal intercourse, as well as a lack of spontaneous erections during the night or early morning.

If you do need to adjust your levels, keep in mind that, unless you have extremely low testosterone, natural techniques to raise your level are more healthful than prescription testosterone shots or creams.

Reference ranges for testosterone are usually grouped by age. These ranges often vary between laboratories, and there is a significant difference between the low value for an older man and the high value for a younger man. Typically, a normal level of free testosterone is between 1.5 to 2.9 percent of the total testosterone value. Consider supplementing if your free testosterone is on the low side and you are having symptoms of low testosterone, even if your total testosterone level is in the normal range. This is particularly true if you are older than sixty. Again, keep in mind that the reference values vary somewhat between laboratories. The determinant should be how you feel in conjunction with the laboratory values. Testosterone levels peak in a man's 20's and then begin a slow decline at about 10% per decade afterward. This can affect a man's muscle strength and exercise tolerance, as well as his libido and erectile function.

ED Can Result From Hormone Imbalances

If your ED problem seems to have hormonal components, i.e. you have symptoms of a low testosterone level the least expensive way to start to resolve it is to supplement with some of the herbs and nutrients listed in this article that have known properties of raising testosterone levels. A good starting point is ginseng, tribulus, and yohimbe. You may also want to try an herbal testosterone enhancing cream like our Testosterone for Men or a combination product.

A second approach, which you can either start with or use if you have no improvement after a month or two, is to have your hormone levels tested with a home saliva test. Such kits are easy to use, requiring that you simply put your saliva sample in a tube and mail it to the testing laboratory.

Saliva testing is the best way to determine free hormone levels. A comprehensive test of five to six hormones usually costs about two hundred dollars. Once you know your hormone levels, you can adjust your diet and supplement with bio-identical hormones to bring your levels back to the appropriate ranges, and depending on how you feel, retest now and then to make sure you are staying in balance.

If a saliva hormone test shows your testosterone and other hormone levels to be normal for your age, your ED problem is most likely not a hormonal issue, and you need to step back and reevaluate the issue.

If, on the other hand, your testosterone level is low, or out of balance related to the other hormones, then your ED issue is most likely due to an age or diet related hormonal imbalance. In this case, supplementing with natural hormones as well as some herbal boosters may alleviate the problem relatively quickly. However, before supplementing with using actual hormones it is imperative that you test your hormone levels..

Testosterone injections usually consist of synthetic testosterone and can cause some serious side effects. They raise testosterone levels far beyond the normal biological ranges almost immediately, which cause the body to completely shut down testosterone production and convert the excess testosterone into other hormones like DHT and estrogen. The net result can be shrinkage of the testicles and breast growth. Transdermal testosterone creams are more easily regulated to achieve a healthy balance.

Saliva vs Blood Testing

Most medical doctors only use blood tests and only test for total testosterone. It is common for older men to have a normal level of total testosterone, but low free testosterone. Only the free component is active. Thus, a value for total testosterone, obtained from a blood sample can be misleading. Also, testosterone is not the only hormone that can affect erectile function when out of balance. High levels of estrogen, unopposed by progesterone or testosterone, as well as low levels of Dehydroepiandrosterone (DHEA) can be directly involved in erectile dysfunction.

DHEA is another important hormone that also begins a gradual decline after age 30 or so at about two percent per year. [31] Low DHEA levels often coexist with low testosterone levels and can affect erectile function. In one study, low levels of DHEA were consistently associated with erectile dysfunction. [32]

Thus, it is very important to test not just testosterone, but the group of critical sex steroid hormones simultaneously. A typical basic saliva test for a man should test at least five of these hormones.

Herbal Supplements That Support General Erectile and Prostate Health

Any man over fifty experiencing erectile dysfunction is most likely also dealing with an unhealthy prostate. This may be in the form of urinary difficulties, benign prostate hyperplasia (BPH), prostatitis or even the beginnings of prostate cancer. Rather than simply try to address the problem of ED, a man would be wise to simultaneously address his prostate health. Often, this will also rectify ED. Below are listed several herbs which can help support good prostate health.

The use of medicinal plants for prostate problems and erectile dysfunction has a history that stretches back several thousand years. In many areas of the world, herbal medicine is the primary—and often the only—treatment for many health conditions. It is interesting to note that approximately 95 percent of pharmaceuticals used in the U.S. and Western Europe are derived from plants.

Professional herbalists often treat erectile dysfunction with several herbs simultaneously. They know that the chemical constituents of many herbs—and foods—act synergistically and often have significantly greater benefit when used together. Synergy between herbs is extremely important and is typically what makes herbal combinations much more powerful. All herbalists know this and use synergy as a more effective way of achieving a successful outcome than extracting specific components of individual herbs. Many of the herbs discussed below have broad beneficial effects that overlap and complement each other.

There is much confusing information about the role of beta-sitosterol in regards to good sexual health. Some "so-called" experts claim that high doses will solve all sexual problems, and several male enhancement products are based on it. However, in nature, nutrients are never found in isolation. Purifying one component of an herb for medicinal purposes is akin to producing a pharmaceutical drug and sometimes results in unintended consequences. Most single element products for resolving erectile dysfunction are quite useless and might even be harmful.

Many manufacturers combine several herbs into a single prostate support product for their synergistic effect. Unfortunately, there are many charlatans that take advantage of the suffering male to hawk products that are at best, useless, and at worst, can be harmful. The best approach for a man suffering from prostate issues or ED is to buy supplements from a reputable professional who deals with male problems regularly.

Saw Palmetto - Traditionally, saw palmetto has been the choice of natural practitioners for treatment for BPH. It is a well-studied herb that has proven value for BPH and may possibly help reduce tumor size in prostate cancer. It has also shown value in treating erectile dysfunction possibly by increasing the health of the prostate. One study, noted that sexual function remained stable during the first year of treatment but improved significantly during the second year. [33] Saw palmetto has very few side effects, and many men report that in addition to helping with erectile function it also enhances libido.

It is important to use a standardized extract of saw palmetto berries. Some supplement manufacturers sell the ground berries of saw palmetto in capsule form. While the berries are indeed healthy, extracts are much more powerful. When you are purchasing a saw palmetto extract, look for the words "standardized to contain 85-95 percent fatty acids and sterols" on the label. The dosage that has proven effective is 320 mg per day divided into two doses of 160 mg or four doses of 80 mg.

While saw palmetto is effective by itself, it is even more effective when used synergistically along with other herbs, like pygeum, nettle and pumpkin seed oils.

Pygeum - Pygeum grows primarily in Africa and is commonly called the African prune tree. Its bark has traditionally been used for the treatment of urinary and prostate problems. A meta-analysis looked at eighteen randomized, controlled trials using extracts of pygeum. These trials included a total of 1562 men with BPH. [34] The review concluded that the studies show pygeum improves the urinary symptoms of BPH with few side effects.

Many studies show that men using pygeum were more than twice as likely to report improvement in overall symptoms. Two European studies treated a total of 348 men with this extract at a dose rate of 50 mg twice daily for two months. [35][36] Significant improvements were noted after the two-month treatment period, particularly in nighttime voiding, a persistently annoying symptom of BPH. Nocturnal frequency was reduced by thirty-two percent, and urinary flow and volume were also significantly improved. Like saw palmetto, the full effects of supplementing with pygeum seem to take effect after a period of use of at least six months.

Pygeum seems to be effective at a dosage of about 100 mg per day. Adverse effects of pygeum are rare and mild. Pygeum does not seem to affect the prostate with quite the same mechanism of action as saw palmetto, although it is similar. Thus, while it is sometimes used alone, more often it is used in combination with saw palmetto and other herbs for the synergistic effect. Unfortunately, as with many herbs, studies are small and limited to short durations due to financial considerations, but the evidence is quite strong that pygeum significantly improves symptoms of BPH. [37][38][39]

Nettle Root (Urtica dioica) - Stinging nettle (or simply nettle) has a long history of therapeutic use for many different health issues. Both the root and the leaves of the plant are used medicinally. The leaves and other above ground parts of the nettle plant have different chemical components from those of the root, and thus different medicinal properties. Both root and leaves have anti-inflammatory properties that make them effective for reducing chronic prostatitis. It also appears that nettle helps reduce the level of sex hormone binding globulin (SHBG) which can help to increase in free testosterone. [40][41]

Nettle root is very effective for treating BPH. Like saw palmetto and pygeum, nettle contains many phytosterols that can help relieve symptoms of prostate dysfunction. Studies have shown that nettle by itself it is not quite as effective as saw palmetto or pygeum in treating BPH, though it is usually combined with both for its synergistic effect.

Nettle has a long history of successful use. It is a highly valued medicinal plant and is used for a variety of conditions. Nettle leaf, used as a tea, has a long and well-documented historical use both as a diuretic and as an anti-inflammatory and it can be quite effective at reducing the joint pain and inflammation associated with arthritis. In some cultures, nettle leaves are cooked and eaten like spinach.

Flower Pollen Extracts - For many years, extracts of flower pollen have been used in Europe to treat BPH and prostatitis. Flower pollen is a concentrated, allergen-free extract of the male seeds of rye grass and various other flowering plants. It is marketed under several different commercial names like Swedish Flower Pollen, Graminex, Cernilton and others. It appears to work via multiple chemical pathways to reduce the severity of both BPH and prostatitis.

It is a well-studied supplement where studies have shown significant statistical improvements in urinary flow, intermittent voiding, dribbling, the number of times one wakes up at night to urinate (nocturia) and urinary retention. [42][43][44][45]

A reduction in symptoms can often occur relatively quickly, but as with most herbal remedies for the prostate, the full effect may not be seen immediately. In a study of seventy-nine patients, 85 percent noted improvements in symptoms within the twelve-week study interval. During this initial phase, no changes were noted in prostate size. However, when the study was extended to one year, twenty-eight patients—approximately 35 percent—showed a mean decrease in prostate volume of about twenty percent. [46] It appears that flower pollen helps the prostate get healthier and while there is no definitive link between BPH and erectile dysfunction, improvement in the health of the prostate always has an impact on erectile function.

The dosage used in most of the studies is about 250 mg of standardized extract per day, divided into two doses.

Garlic - Garlic is one of several edible plants of the genus allium in the lily family. It has been used both as food and medicine for thousands of years in virtually every culture. It is known to reduce blood pressure and cholesterol levels and increase blood circulation in both animals and humans. As mentioned earlier in this article, any improvement in blood circulation is tantamount to an improvement in resolving erectile dysfunction. Garlic appears to help increase nitric oxide levels allowing better erections.

Garlic can be consumed in many ways. You can mix it with almost any food, and it can be eaten cooked or raw. If you do not like Garlic, you can purchase a condensed supplement. Regardless of how you take it, adding garlic and the other allium vegetables to your diet on a regular basis can improve your health dramatically.

Herbs That Can Beat ED

Above we discussed some herbs that can help with general health. Often, improving overall health with a better diet and some herbs is enough to restore libido and help resolve erectile dysfunction. For some men however, the problem is more intense and may need additional prodding.

As we have discussed, hormone balance is critical to overall prostate health as well as sexual function. Many of the herbs discussed below work by helping the body balance hormone levels that have gone astray.

Unfortunately, in the area of sexual dysfunction, there is much misleading information. This is particularly true for information on the Internet where supplement sellers can reach many men, and make almost any claim they want with little proof of efficacy. As a result, many items sold today for prostate or sexual problems have little basis for recommending them other than the claims of the manufacturer or his agent. On the other hand, some herbs and nutritional items have considerable historical and anecdotal evidence, and a growing number have clinical evidence supporting their benefits.

Supplement manufacturers are quick to exploit any positive link to their products, and the pharmaceutical industry is also quick to promote negative information for natural items. A person in the middle, tying to sift through all the conflicting information, has a tough task indeed. The number of studies done in the United States on herbal remedies is far behind the rest of the world, but the gap appears to be closing. Herbal remedies are becoming more popular in the U.S., and as a result, they are gathering more attention from researchers. While much of the herbal world is still based on folklore and historical use, more clinical studies are being done on natural preparations. In addition, some medical doctors are starting to realize the value of herbal remedies and prescribe them.

An erection is a complex event that requires the cooperation of many body systems. As a man becomes sexually aroused, nerve signals cause an increase in a chemical called nitric oxide (NO) in the genital area. This is the primary agent that begins a cascade of chemical actions that then result in an erection. Without nitric oxide, it would be impossible to produce an erection.

A thin layer of specialized cells called the endothelium lines the inside of all blood vessels in the body. This tissue controls constriction or dilation of blood vessels. Dysfunction in this tissue is linked to several chronic conditions, including, but not limited to, erectile dysfunction, heart disease, and atherosclerosis. [47] One of the main indicators of endothelial dysfunction is a diminished level of nitric oxide. Improving endothelial function via exercise or nutritional and/or herbal supplements can go a long way towards reducing the severity of erectile dysfunction and many other problems.

**Ginkgo** Traditional Chinese herbalists have used Ginkgo for many years. It is well researched and has become one of the top selling medicinal herbs worldwide. Ginkgo's proven effectiveness in improving blood circulation throughout the body also makes it a useful herb for overcoming the circulation problems inherent with erectile dysfunction.

Ginkgo is known to improve blood circulation throughout the body. Extracts of Ginkgo are included in many men's health supplements for its ability to promote healthy circulation.

In Europe, ginkgo is used for treating many different problems including impaired memory, tinnitus (ringing in the ears), and dizziness, all of which can be caused by insufficient blood flow to the brain. Ginkgo is generally regarded as extremely safe, has few side effects, and can be take for long periods of time. [48] One of gingko's effects is to thin the blood, so it should not be taken by anyone who is anticipating surgery in the immediate future, or is using prescription blood-thinning medication.

Gingko is a bulky herb. It takes a lot of leaf to make a useful amount. Typical gingko preparations are concentrated 50:1 extracts, meaning that it takes fifty ounces of leaf to produce one ounce of product. Use only gingko produced by a reputable manufacturer that is at least a 50:1 extract and standardized to contain at least twenty-four percent flavonglycosides and six percent terpene lactones. A typical dosage of such an extract is 120 mg per day divided into two or four doses.

Ginseng – This Asian herb has an extensive reputation as an aphrodisiac and sexual tonic. Studies have shown it to be effective in modulating blood pressure, enhancing immune response, raising libido and generally helping improve health. There are different varieties with similar properties, but the Asian (sometimes called Korean) red panex ginseng has the most significant value for men with sexual dysfunction.

Panex ginseng has been shown in several studies of both animals and humans to promote increased sperm production, raise testosterone levels, and enhance erectile capacity. [49] [50] There is also some anecdotal evidence that it lowers the orgasmic threshold, making it easier for one to have an orgasm. It is considered to be quite safe.

Ginseng does not have as strong an effect on erectile dysfunction as yohimbe. Its main effect appears to be due to its influence on related systems. Since ginseng can act as a stimulant, some users may notice side effects. Most notably, these are sleep problems or anxiety, and, with higher doses, occasional heart palpitations.

When purchasing ginseng, select only Korean (Asian) red ginseng root extract standardized to provide 5 percent ginsenosides. Typical capsule sizes available vary from 100 to 400 mg. Keep in mind that individuals may respond differently to ginseng. It may work well for one person, but another might experience side effects. It is best to start with a low dose and watch for adverse effects. Typical dosage is about 300 to 1000 mg per day, but many individuals use more. Research studies have used up to 4,500 mg per day in test subjects without ill effects. Doses higher than typical should be used only under the direction of a health professional.

Yohimbe - One of the most studied herbs for erectile dysfunction is Yohimbe. Its active ingredient is an alkaloid extracted from the bark known as yohimbine hydrochloride, or yohimbine. It was the first item approved for use by the FDA for erectile dysfunction. Yohimbine is available only as a prescription medicine. Standard extracts of the bark however, also contain yohimbine and are available from Natural Health Practitioners.

Yohimbe's action is similar to other erectile dysfunction drugs currently available by prescription. It increases blood flow to the erectile tissue of the penis. Yohimbe differs from other impotence drugs in that it also tends to increase testosterone levels and thereby libido. Studies have confirmed that yohimbe is effective for reducing erectile dysfunction in up to 55 percent of men. [51][52][53] While this level of effectiveness is somewhat lower than that of other erectile dysfunction drugs, considering that yohimbe is a natural rather than synthetic agent, and also tends to increase libido, possibly via an increase in testosterone levels, it is worthwhile to consider it as a first line treatment, especially for men with less severe problems.

There has been some question as to the safety of yohimbe when used directly from the bark, and some experts have cautioned of dangerous side effects. [54][55][56] The most serious side effects the studies noted were a slight elevation of blood pressure and anxiety levels in some men. Other side effects appear to be minimal. If you are in the percentile of men for whom yohimbe is effective, you probably will not suffer any significant side effects. However, if you are prone to have high blood pressure, or you suffer from serious depression, panic attacks or anxiety, it is wise not to use yohimbe, since it could make such problems worse.

The actual amount of yohimbine and potency of an extract depends on how the yohimbe bark is processed and on the manufacturer's integrity. One study of commercial yohimbe supplements found that many contain little or no yohimbine. [57] Stick to a well-known manufacturer's product, or buy from a well-known natural health practitioner that researches sources. Supplements should contain a standardized extract of yohimbe bark yielding at least two, but no more than ten mg of yohimbines.

Maca - Maca is a cruciferous vegetable that produces a root similar to a turnip or potato and is a staple and versatile food product. It grows in Peru and Peruvians use it as Americans use potatoes and also to make cookies, cakes, chips, and various flavored drinks. Maca is an important food in the Peruvian diet with a rich nutrient profile. Its reputation comes from a history of folklore of several hundred years. Most supplements for erectile dysfunction have a direct effect on the mechanism that produces an erection. They either increase the chemical messengers that produce an erection or decrease those that prevent it. For some, the messenger is nitric oxide. For others, it is androgen hormones like testosterone. Maca is a notable exception. Clinical studies have shown that maca has virtually no effect on testosterone and the other sex steroid hormones. [58] It also does not appear to have any effect on nitric oxide levels. However, many recent clinical studies on maca in both animals and adult men seem to agree that the herb increases sexual drive and ability. In animal studies, rats fed maca were observed to have a significantly greater sexual response. [59][60][61]

As a food, Maca is loaded with nutrients. It is quite possible its reported benefits are due to its high concentration of protein, amino acids, phytosterols, and other nutrients. Maca is also high in arginine, an essential amino acid involved in sexual functioning.

Since maca is a known food staple with a fabulous nutrient profile, it is unlikely that it will do any harm. Considering that it is relatively inexpensive and safe, it is certainly worth a try.

Macu is used in many male enhancement supplements in such small quantities that there is little chance it will be of any help. The best way to use it is as a bulk powdered herb. You can use the powder in a beverage, or sprinkle it on food.

Horny Goat Weed - Aside from the provocative name, horny goat weed has a reputation that stretches back more than 2000 years. In

Chinese medicine, it is known as Yin Yang Huo and it is used for treating disorders of the kidneys and liver as well as sexual dysfunction.

Chinese herbalists believe it helps the body restore levels of testosterone—particularly free testosterone—and thyroid hormones. [62] Horny goat weed also appears to cause blood vessels and capillaries to dilate, thus increasing blood flow to the sexual organs. One study was done on mice with erectile dysfunction induced by poor arterial circulation. The study concluded that it significantly improved erectile function and nitric oxide levels in the erectile tissue of the tested mice. [63]

As with Maca, Horny Goat Weed is an ingredient in most male enhancement supplements. Unfortunately, many manufacturers put such small quantities in their products that they are unlikely to have any noticeable effect on male performance.

A typical dose should be 500 mg two to four times daily of an extract standardized to contain at least 10 percent icariins.

Tribulus or Puncture Vine- Tribulus has been used for hundreds of years as a treatment for both male and female sexual problems and has a reputation among body-builders for building muscle. In many countries it is widely used by athletes. In India, tribulus is used in ayurveda, the ancient Hindu science of health and medicine, as both a tonic and aphrodisiac.

Tribulus does seem to enhance libido by promoting a slight increase in testosterone by a different path then hormonal precursors like DHEA and androstenedione.

While there is an abundance of information about tribulus on the Internet, few studies have been published. In its favor, tribulus contains phyto-chemicals called steroidal furostanol saponins, or more simply saponins. One of them, called "protodioscin" is known to improve sexual desire and enhance erection. Studies in animals and humans have shown that protodioscin increases levels of both testosterone and DHEA.

[64][65] Other saponins also appear to be active in tribulus and may account for some of its activity. Tribulus is a complex herb that seems to have interesting effects on the body. New saponins recently discovered may be found to be as, or more active, than protodioscin regarding libido enhancement or erectile function. [66][67]

There are no reported problems with using tribulus, and it does not appear to have any serious side effects. Even so, tribulus has been known to have toxic effects on sheep. If you decide to try it, start with a low dose and gradually increase it watching for any adverse effects. Purchase only an extract from a reputable manufacturer, standardized to contain at least 20 percent protodioscin, and a minimum of 30 to 40 percent steroidal saponins (furostanol). A typical dosage is 750-1500 mg daily, divided into three doses at mealtimes.

The Hype About Male Enhancement/ED Products

There are many herbs used in male sexual enhancement products. In this book, I have listed several of the most common, and more importantly, well-studies herbal and nutritional items.

Unfortunately, most male sexual enhancement products have nothing more going for them than the excitement and imagination of those producing them. Few have any scientific basis for their use. This is not to say that all of these commercial products are useless, but just that there is not much data supporting them.

I have personally researched many of the products advertised on late night T.V. for both ingredients, and efficacy. Manufacturers have asked me to support their products on my website, which I will be happy to do, if they provide me with detailed ingredients lists, safety analysis, and enough samples to actually test the items. So far, manufacturers have only provided lots of paperwork "propaganda" and advertising information. The only product that a manufacturer actually provided some samples of, failed miserably.

As of this writing, I have seen some heavy advertising for a sexual enhancement product that is hyped to make every man into a "super-stud". It didn't take much research to realize that the only active ingredient in this product was the common amino acid L-Carnitine. While L-Carnitine can certainly help the overall health of a man suffering from ED, there is very little science that justifies it having more than a minimal effect on resolving ED. But, you would never know that from their advertisements, and I'll bet they have sold lots of product to some very disappointed men!

Synergy

I have mentioned synergy many times in this book. In a recent well-designed study, a combination of arginine and yohimbine was compared with yohimbine alone in a group of forty-five men. [68] Patients with mild to moderate ED responded better to the combination of arginine and yohimbe than to yohimbe alone, and both groups did better than a placebo group. This synergistic effect often occurs with other herbs and vitamins as well.

You may find that a combination of one or more of the items discussed here may be more helpful than any single item taken alone. Another study of a product containing three grams of arginine, along with ginseng (200 mg), ginkgo (50 mg), and several other vitamins and minerals, reported that 88.9 percent of the participants improved their ability to maintain an erection during sexual intercourse after four weeks using the product. No significant side effects were reported. [69]

Things to Avoid

In this book, I have discussed several nutrients and herbs that are beneficial for a man with ED. However, there are also some items that can worsen the situation.

__Licorice__ — This herb, an ingredient in many candies, flavoring agents, breath fresheners, over the counter remedies, and even some male sexual enhancement products, can cause problems when consumed regularly or in large quantities. Licorice contains a chemical called glycyrrhizin that can deplete the body's potassium, cause water retention, and lead to high blood pressure. This can happen with as little as five to seven grams of licorice root per day on a regular basis. Of additional concern to a man with ED is that licorice has been reported to lower testosterone levels. [70] This is certainly not what a man suffering from ED wants.

If you currently consume licorice and you suffer from erectile dysfunction, it would be wise for you to curtail licorice consumption for several months to see if your symptoms improve. Fortunately, it appears that the effect licorice has on the body is reversed when consumption of it is eliminated. In any event, it is probably wise to avoid any more than occasional use of licorice, especially if you suffer from erectile dysfunction or hypertension.

__Fatty Meals__ —High fat meals, particularly those high in animal fat, lead to many problems with one's health. Often a man will consume a large meal and later finds that an attempt at sexual intercourse results in failure. When your body is busy digesting a heavy meal, it is not going to be able to divert a significant amount of blood from the digestion process to the penis. The solution is simple—eat a lighter meal or wait longer to digest a heavier one before attempting sexual activity.

__Medications__ —Many prescription drugs, particularly antidepressants, blood pressure medications and pain relievers, have a long history of causing sexual problems, both by reducing libido and causing erectile dysfunction. This is very well known and has been documented in clinical studies. If you are on antidepressants and you suffer from erectile dysfunction, consult with your doctor about possibly switching to a different drug or using some of the herbs suggested in this book to offset the side effects.

In addition, some commonly used pain relievers, known as NSAIDs (nonsteroidal anti-inflammatory drugs) like ibuprofen or naproxen, as well as the prescription drug Celebrex, can cause irritation and/or urinary retention. In a Dutch study men that were actively using NSAIDs had double the risk of developing acute urinary retention.[71] It is well known that several types of cold remedies containing anti-histamines can cause severe prostate irritation, particularly when used by men with BPH.

Marijuana — While not generally as dangerous as some of the other illicit drugs, marijuana has produced controversial results when studied for its effects on sexual functioning. Some studies have shown it to lower testosterone and other androgen levels while others have shown it to have little effect. In small doses it seems to have a relaxing effect which would be conducive to better sex. However, Marijuana smokers inhale carcinogens with the smoke just like tobacco smokers. A recent study implicated it as a causative factor for the same kind of cancers caused by tobacco. [72] Thus, it is prudent to avoid it.

Other Illicit Drugs — Most of the other illicit drugs have a clear history of producing addiction and inhibiting sexual drive and ability. Some—like cocaine—produce an initial euphoria that may lead to heightened sexual performance for a short while. However, with continued use the euphoria fades, and sexual ability is crippled. Other drugs—like those in the opiate family, (heroin, morphine, methadone, etc.), are central nervous system depressants and typically inhibit both sexual desire and ability almost immediately. With their continued use the effect tends to multiply, eventually resulting in an almost complete lack of libido and total or near total impotence. If you value your sex life, do not mess with illicit drugs!

If Supplements Don't Work

There are times, of course, when supplements do not work, even after they are given sufficient trial time. This leaves a man with little other recourse than to try a medical approach. There are several medical approaches to treating ED. Many men suffer from Erectile Dysfunction after prostate or other pelvic surgery. This is sometimes temporary and other times permanent, and unfortunately, there is no way to tell if it will be temporary or not.

Others suffer from ED due to concurrent illnesses like diabetes, which often desensitizes the erectile nerves to a point where they no longer function, and spinal or other injuries can cause permanent ED.

Several treatments are discussed below. Vacuum Erection Devices and Penile Implants are mechanical solutions. The Vacuum Erection Device is non-invasive and can allow a man to get an erection at will. Being non-invasive, it can be easily used for penile rehabilitation after prostate or other pelvic surgery, and can be stopped at any time. It can be quite valuable for a man who has had prostate or pelvic surgery and is temporarily impotent. It can also be quite valuable for permanent ED, since it will usually produce a usable erection as long as the penis has not been physically damaged. A Penile Implant is a permanent surgical replacement of the erectile channels, thus, it is an invasive, non-reversible procedure. Injectable and implantable drugs can also help, but again they suffer from serious side effects.

Regardless of what the source of your ED is, you can take comfort in the fact that you can probably restore some degree of function and have a reasonable amount of sexual satisfaction using one or more of the techniques or devices below.

Oral Drugs for ED

Some of these, like the FDA approved prescription ED drugs have a history of being effective, albeit they can cause undesirable side effects for many men. However, they rarely work if the erectile nerves are damaged due to surgery or injury. Many men, no doubt influenced by constant bombardment of ED drug advertisements, view it as a simple problem that can (or should) be quickly remedied with a prescription drug. Unfortunately, some of their overworked doctors simply do not take the time to evaluate all their risk factors before reaching for a prescription pad.

While treating ED with medication typically results in a happy patient, it does little to correct underlying circulation problems which are then allowed to progress unchecked. Prescribing an ED drug without dealing with such underlying vascular issues is blindly treating a symptom while ignoring the real problem. Eventually, the erectile dysfunction may be of little concern when a man begins to suffer from serious vascular problems such as angina, a coronary event, or a stroke.

If you suffered from erectile dysfunction back in the days before the FDA approved erectile dysfunction drugs you had no choice but to use vitamins, herbs, and lifestyle changes to regain function. Today, a man doesn't have to work that hard. A quick trip to the doctor will usually result in a prescription for one of the three, and in most cases, the *symptoms* of impotence will be resolved.

Any man who feels this is the best course of action is fooling himself in a big way! ED drugs are not risk-free. Side effects of these drugs can include eye problems, epileptic seizures, convulsions and sleep apnea. Carefully worded warnings are also in the literature that comes with the drug. [73] [74] [75] [76] [77]

If you are willing to accept the risks, you can use an ED drug to temporarily alleviate the immediate problem. However, this should be considered only as a temporary solution. In that case, Cialis appears to have a profile that is least likely to cause disturbances with the retina of the eye.[78]

ED drugs cause a temporary increase in blood flow, resulting in a firmer erection. However, they do not clear clogged arteries, nor do they correct hormone levels. Thus, while they provide effective short-term relief from symptoms, they do little to rectify any underlying conditions. A permanent solution for erectile dysfunction is best achieved by addressing the problem at its source through lifestyle changes and improvement of overall health.

Other Drug Treatments

Aside from the oral FDA approved ED drugs, there are several non-oral methods of resolving ED. Each of these depends on introducing Prostaglandin (PGE-1) with or without other chemicals into the corpus cavernousum of the penis. These are the two vein like tubes that run the length of the penis from the base to its head. When a man is aroused, PGE-1 is released causing the corpus cavernosum to fill with blood and produce an erection. For most men, PGE-1, when introduced into the corpus cavernosum, will reliably produce an erection every time.

There are three drugs commonly used for this purpose: Prostaglandin, Papaverine and Phentolamine. Each of these is a vasodilator that helps increase blood flow into the corpus cavernosum, with Prostaglandin being the strongest and most widely used. In the U.S., these medications require a valid prescription from a licensed medical practitioner and are sometimes mixed together and called Trimix.

Caution: Some Men's clinics sell customized prescriptions of Trimix to their clients at exorbitant prices. If you decide to try Trimix injections, consult with a reputable urologist and compounding pharmacy. A five ml vial of Trimix typically costs about $100 to $150.

There are several ways to introduce the drugs into the penis. The most direct approach is intracavernous injection therapy or simply injection therapy. In this process the single or combined drug mix is injected directly into the side of the penis and into the cavernosa tissue of the penis. This causes the smooth muscles of the penis to relax, thus allowing increased blood flow into the penis. A erection is produced with a few minutes and can last for 1-2 hours. The disadvantage of this technique is that the man must give himself an injection directly into his penis before sex, and apply pressure to the injection site for a few minutes, which is not always conducive to a relaxed atmosphere for sex. One of the side effects of this medication is an increased risk of priaprism, an undesired erection that lasts several hours and can permanently damage the penis if not treated immediately. It can also exacerbate Peyronie's disease (curvature of the penis on erection). Other side effects include needle damage at the injection site, hematoma and development of scar tissue in the penis

Most men that use this technique become comfortable with it after their initial hesitancy. The cost of using a Trimix injection depends on the patient's prescription concentration but typically ranges between $3 and $10 per injection.

Trimix is also be supplied in Gel form. In this case, a specialized applicator is provided to insert the gel into the urethra. This method is not in wide use due to its high cost and low efficacy. The typical cost for six applicators is nearly $200 US, making a single erection cost about $33. Using the applicator per the instructions often results in loss of the gel, so, in reality, the actual cost can be considerably higher.

Another system, called Medicated Urethral System for Erection (MUSE), is also in use by some urologists. It consists of a tablet of Alprostadil (PGE-1) that is inserted through the tip of the penis using a special insertion device packaged with the drug. The tablet slowly dissolves in the urethra releasing the PGE-1 chemical for absorption into the corpus cavernosum. When properly inserted, it can result in a usable erection within 10-15 minutes. It does not work for all men and reports of efficacy vary widely from less than 10% to over 60%. Many men stop using it due to its unreliability and high cost.

Another method, similar to the MUSE and Trimix Gel method above is to use Misoprostol (a synthetic PGE-1) inserted in liquid form into the urethra. This method requires that the user dissolve the misoprostol tablet in water, place a restrictive band on the head of his penis, and then insert, via an eyedropper or similar device, a measured solution of the chemical into his urethra Like the MUSE method above, this depends on the PGE-1 chemical being absorbed into the corpus cavernosum through the urethra. However, as long as the restrictive ring on the penis is tight enough to eliminate leakage of the inserted solution, this method can be quite effective. It typically results in an erection within 10-15 minutes, at which time the restrictive ring is removed. The erection typically lasts about an hour or a little more. This method is by far the least expensive of the above options. Cost of an erection can range between $2 and $4

Each of these techniques can help men that have nerve damage due to non-nerve-sparing pelvic surgery or radical prostatectomy. Because these drugs do not depend on functional erectile nerves they can also help men with nerve damage that does not respond to other ED drugs.

Injection therapy appears to be more effective than the other methods and has a success rate of close to 90%, but a high percentage of men stop using it within a few months.

Some men have found that using the last method above with a low dose of misoprostol and then enhancing their erection afterward with a Vacuum Erection Device can improve both their performance and satisfaction

Vacuum Erection Devices

Vacuum Erection Devices (VED's) are one of the most popular solutions to the problem of ED. They are a safe and effective alternative to implant surgery or oral medication, especially for a man who is suffering temporary ED due to illness or surgery. VED's are very affordable and satisfaction rates are high.

A vacuum erection device (VED), sometimes called a penis pump uses a small pump or motor to create a vacuum on the penis. This pulls blood into the erectile chambers of the penis causing it to become erect. The erection is then maintained by placing a constricting ring at the base of the penis.

VED's have proven to be very useful for a man who's ED is due to prostate or pelvic surgery. The devices produce a near normal erection and are also sometimes used for penile rehabilitation and to prevent prenile shrinkage due to atrophy of the penile tissues.

Prostate surgery—even the nerve sparing kind—often causes the erectile nerves to go into shock—a condition known as neuroplaxia. While the nerves often recover spontaneously, the process of recovery might take up to two years. During this time, the lack of all erections may cause penile tissue to become undernourished and shrink, leaving the man with a far smaller penis than before the surgery, and diminished erectile function. VED's are useful for men that are motivated to resume sexual activity as soon as possible after surgery as well as men who want to maximize the chance of regaining normal erectile function and maintaining penile length.

Vacuum Erection devices are useful for men that cannot get a useable erection, men whose erection does not last long enough for vaginal penetration, or to help men with premature ejaculation maintain an erection after ejaculation. They can also help with penile rehabilitation after surgery. By forcing blood into the penis daily—creating one or more erections and holding them for about 10 minutes—they simulate the natural bodily action that occurs with normal nocturnal erections. Studies have shown that this may help preserve penile length and hasten recovery of sexual function after surgery.

Using a VED is a matter of choice and finances. Many men find that a VED is far less expensive—over the long range—than prescription ED medications, which are typically not covered by medical insurance, and can cost more than $10 per pill.

Note that these units provide a mechanical fix only. They will not restore your sex drive or desire but they can improve your sexual ability simply by generating a usable erection.

Nerve Stimulation for Erectile Dysfunction

Transcutaneous electrical nerve stimulation (TENS) is used for many degenerative conditions both to accelerate nerve regeneratation and treat pain. TENS units have proven useful to help with conditions like diabetic polyneuropathy. This disease occurs in diabetics—particularly men—and causes painful damage, malfunction and eventual destruction of nerve cells, usually in the toes and feet. The word polyneuropathy literally means damage to many nerves. The disease is caused by an increased in inflammation due to the high levels of blood glucose having a damaging effect on both nerves fibers and small blood vessels in various parts of the body. In diabetic polyneuropathy, the damage is primarily in the feet and hands, but often also includes erectile and penile nerves. It is essentially, a circulatory disorder. The probability of the disorder progressing increases with age.

Most men that suffer from erectile dysfunction have circulatory disorders similar to that mentioned above for the very same reasons. Risk factors include lack of exercise, poor diet, obesity, atherosclerosis, high blood pressure, heavy alcohol use, smoking and diabetes. All of these produce chronic circulatory problems particularly in diabetics, and many cases result in erectile dysfunction, as well as other circulatory disorders. These disorders tend to develop slowly over time, and often do not get much attention until they become chronic or have reached a critical stage.

Although there is little research on use of a TENS machine for ED, it is well known that electrical currents passed through the skin (transcutaneous) stimulate nerves. Some men have experimented with TENS therapy for erectile dysfunction and claim some success, but I could not find any actual research studies. However, TENS therapy has been used successfully for chronic pain for many years. While it is mostly used to help alleviate pain, it is well-recognized that such therapy also leads to an increase in blood flow in the treated area. Again, anything that increases blood circulation to the penis also brings it additional nutrients and helps produce recovery.

Obtaining and using a TENS machine is easy. Machines are inexpensive and are now available for over-the-counter purchase without a prescription. Units are typically battery powered and provided with adhesive electrodes that are placed directly on the skin, producing a tingling sensation when turned on. The electrical impulses travel through the electrodes and the skin, reaching and stimulating the nerves.

Most TENS devices have a method for controlling the pulse frequency and intensity. The little research I could find on this seems to indicate that low frequencies, in the order of 10 Hz or less tend to stimulate blood circulation in the treated area. At higher frequencies and amplitude, the device tends to stimulate muscle contraction. This may also be of use in treating erectile dysfunction.

Since there is little research on using a TENS unit for ED, any man that wishes to try it is completely on his own. If misused, a TENS unit could possibly cause skin irritation or burns, especially if used at high intensity. However, since the machines are quite inexpensive, and that most experts consider them to be safe, a man with a careful and experimental nature might find one to be helpful for his ED.

Shock Wave Treatment

High intensity extracorporeal shock wave treatment (ESWT) is a medical procedure where a high-intensity sonic pulse is applied outside of the body (extracorporeal) but focused on an internal target. This procedure (known as lithotripsy) has been used successfully for many years to break up stones in the kidney, bladder, or the ureters that carry urine from your kidneys to your bladder. High-Intensity ESWL is one of the least invasive methods for stone treatment.

Similarly, medium intensity shock waves are used to reduce inflammation and to aid healing in a variety of orthopedic conditions; most notably in helping fractured bones heal. The latest generation machines use an acoustic lens that functions much like an optical lens to focus the shock wave allowing more precise aiming of the shock wave.

High and medium intensity ESWL are generally accepted and approved procedures, but in a new application of this technology, researchers have begun developing and testing low-intensity ESWL for treatment of erectile dysfunction with good results. [79] [80][81]

The theory about how ESWT helps promote healing rests on the idea that the repetitive shock wave induces micro-trauma to the affected area. This micro-trauma causes microscopic damage to muscle fibers. The body responds by producing and increasing new blood flow (neo-vascularization) into the area, replacing the damaged muscle tissue and adding to it. This is what causes increase muscle size through weight training. Also, the increased blood flow results in more nutrients being delivered to the damaged tissue promoting tissue healing and recovery. [82]

ESWT uses essentially the same theory for restoring erectile tissue, i.e., long-term training causes trauma to the treated area, which then results in neo-vascularization. This increase in size and capability of the erectile tissue helps it withstand additional stress and function better.

The low intensity shock waves are about 10% of those used to destroy kidney stones, and are delivered to the corpus cavernosa of the penis through a specially designed shock-wave applicator.

Erectile Dysfunction is caused by many different conditions. However, the most prevalent cause in aging men is due to circulation problems. As I mention in many sections of this book, anything that increases circulation in the body will tend to help reduce erectile dysfunction. Increasing blood flow and strengthening erectile muscles and surrounding areas of the penis is certainly an interesting approach to solving ED.

Recently, ESWT has become available at some Men's clinics throughout to US. Be careful though, many of these so called "Clinics" are geared more to take your money than resolve your problem. A typical cost appears to range from about $300 to $600 per treatment. Since, the recommendation is a minimum of six treatments, this can be a rather costly experience.

Currently, use of ESWT seems to be expanding to many medical disciplines, the most promising of which appear to be accelerated wound healing and the treatment of ED. The ESWT technology is approved in the US by the Food and Drug Administration (FDA) for treatment of a several conditions and several doctors and clinics are using it for treating conditions like ED

Low intensity ESWT is a very promising treatment method, with few adverse effects, that may be able to achieve the restoration of natural erectile function without the use of drugs.

Penile Implants

This is the absolute last resort for resolving erectile dysfunction. It requires a 1-2 hour surgery, and is generally not reversible. There are two types of penile implants; a semi-rigid rod implant, and inflatable implants.

The semi-rigid rods are implanted in the corpora cavernosum of the penis, (the chambers that fill with blood during an erection) and the penis is simply bent up for sexual use or down for normal living. This of course maintains the penis in sort of a semi-erect state all the time, and there is no change in length or girth regardless of the position of the semi-rigid rods. It requires the least amount of surgery, and thus, is the least expensive and also the least natural of the penile implants.

Inflatable penis implants are more commonly used and considered more effective. The implants consist of two inflatable tubes that are inserted into the corpora cavernosum of the penis. These tubes connect to a saline-filled reservoir that is manually pumped by the man to fill the implants and achieve an erection on demand. Filling of the implants with saline solution is very similar to the action of a natural erection and like a natural erection, it causes an increase in both length and girth of the penis from the flaccid state. However, the increase is limited to roughly the same size the man had before the procedure.

Depending on the procedure chosen, the manual pump and reservoir can be located either in the scrotum or implanted in the abdominal wall. Prior to sexual activity, the man squeezes the pump, which fills the inflatable implants in the penis with the saline solution from the reservoir, producing an erection. When sexual activity is complete, he presses a release button on the reservoir, allowing the implants to deflate, and the penis returns to its pre-erect size and hardness.

The surgery requires opening the base of the penis or scrotum to implant the rods or inflatable implants, and has a recovery time of about

4-6 weeks. As with all surgery, there is a risk of infection or complications. Insurance may or may not cover the procedure. It should also be noted that penile implants do not cause expansion of the tip of the penis (the glans), thus, the erection produced does not quite expand this area, resulting in a somewhat different appearance than a normal erection.

Satisfaction with these procedures varies from doctor to doctor and patient to patient. The skills of the doctor is also a strong determinant of patient satisfaction, as well as options for the type of implant. Patient satisfaction seems to be highest with the inflatable implant with an abdominally implanted reservoir. Since the reservoir is larger, it holds more fluid, thus more fluid can be transferred to the penis to produce a harder erection.

This should be considered to be a non-reversible procedure with considerable risks. It behooves any man about to try it to check out all the other non-invasive or minimally invasive techniques for resolving ED before going to this level. Before proceeding with an implant, it is also wise to communicate with other men who have had the procedure, check out the surgeon you are considering—and get references from his patients. [83]

Conclusion and Summary

Unfortunately, while a tremendous amount of study has been devoted to resolving erectile dysfunction with medications and medical techniques, there are few controlled scientific studies on the effects of natural substances to resolve the problem. To compound the problem, much of the research on natural products is done outside the United States, preventing widespread knowledge in this country due to language problems and inaccessibility of some publications. Fortunately, the Internet and popular search engines like Google have now matured to the point where such information is readily available even when written in a foreign language.

Recognizing that ED is a serious physical problem, and one that can severely affect quality of life as well as that of your relationship partner, I have listed many techniques in this book that may help resolve the issue. Some of these natural; re; vitamins, herbs, lifestyle, and hormone balancing, some non-invasive medical; re: vacuum erection devices; some are drug solutions; re: FDA approved ED drugs, and some invasive medical procedures; re: penile implants.

If a man with ED approaches his problem scientifically, he should first determine the approximate cause of his ED. The first part of this book can help you do that. Once a probable cause is determined, use the information in part 2 to help resolve the issue. Keep in mind that most natural solutions might take a few months to affect any real help. Approved ED drugs, if they work for you, can be a temporary and instant solution, as can a vacuum erection device. I have seen many men achieve a high degree of satisfaction combining a vacuum erection device with herbal remedies and/or prescription ED drugs.

In any event, recognize that there is no such thing as a *"one size fits all"* approach to this sort of problem. Also, keep in mind that the preponderance of male sexual supplements heavily advertised (especially on late night T.V.) are mostly useless.

However, with patience and a little experimentation, you can be assured that you can resolve your Erectile Dysfunction. It may take a while, but it *will* happen!

References:

[1] Bacon, C., et al. Sexual Function in Men Older Than 50 Years of Age: Results from the Health Professionals Follow-up Study. *Annals of Internal Medicine,* Vol. 139, No. 3:161-168, Aug. 2003.

[2] Bonierbale, M.; et al, The ELIXIR study: evaluation of sexual dysfunction in 4557 depressed patients in France *Current Medical Research and Opinion,* Vol. 19, No. 2:114-124, March 2003.

[3] Gregorian, R.,. et al. Antidepressant-induced sexual dysfunction. *The Annals of Pharmacotherapy,* Vol. 36, No. 10:1577-89. Oct. 2002.

[4] Waldinger, M., et al, Effect of SSRI Antidepressants on Ejaculation: A Double-Blind, Randomized, Placebo-Controlled Study With Fluoxetine, Fluvoxamine, Paroxetine, and Sertraline. *Journal of Clinical Psychopharmacology,* Vol. 18, No. 4:274-281, Aug. 1998.

[5] Nurnberg, H., Managing Treatment-Emergent Sexual Dysfunction Associated with Serotonergic Antidepressants: Before and After Sildenafil. *Journal of Psychiatric Practice,* Vol. 7, No. 2:92-108, March 2001.

[6] Labbate, L., et al. Antidepressant-related erectile dysfunction: management via avoidance, switching antidepressants, antidotes, and adaptation. *The Journal of Clinical Psychiatry,* Vol. 64, No. 10:11-9, Aug. 2003.

[7] Kantor, J., et al. Prevalence of Erectile Dysfunction and Active Depression: An Analytic Cross-Sectional Study of General Medical Patients. *American Journal of Epidemiology,* Vol. 156, No. 11, Dec. 2002.

[8] Kirby, M., et al, Is erectile dysfunction a marker for cardiovascular disease? *International Journal of Clinical Practice,* Vol. 55, No.9:614-618,. Nov. 2001.

[9] Tomeo, A., et al. Antioxidant effects of tocotrienols in patients with hyperlipidemia and carotid stenosis. *Lipids,* Vol. 30, No. 12:1179-83, Dec 1995.

[10] Qureshi, A., Lowering of serum cholesterol in hypercholesterolemic humans by tocotrienols. *American Journal of Clinical Nutrition*, Vol. 53, 1021S-1026S, 1991.

[11] Chandan, K., Tocotrienol: The Natural Vitamin E to Defend the Nervous System. *Annals of the New York Academy of Sciences*, Vol. 1031: 127–142, Dec. 2004.

[12] Schleithoff, S., et al. Vitamin D supplementation improves cytokine profiles in patients with congestive heart failure: a double-blind, randomized, placebo-controlled trial. *American Journal of Clinical Nutrition*, Vol. 83, No. 4:754-759, April 2006.

[13] Cigolini, M., et al. Serum 25-Hydroxyvitamin D3 Concentrations and Prevalence of Cardiovascular Disease Among Type 2 Diabetic Patients. *Diabetes Care*, Vol. 29:722-724, March 2006.

[14] National Institutes of Health, Dietary Supplement Fact Sheet: Vitamin D, Office of Dietary Supplements, NIH Clinical Center.

[15] Rostand, S., et al. Ultraviolet light may contribute to geographic and racial blood pressure differences. *Hypertension*, Vol. 30, No. 2:150-156, Aug. 1997.

[16] Zittermann, A., et al. Putting cardiovascular disease and vitamin D insufficiency into perspective. *British Journal of Nutrition*, Vol. 94, No. 4:483-492, Oct. 2005.

[17] Skinner, H., el al. Vitamin D Intake and the Risk for Pancreatic Cancer in Two Cohort Studies. *Cancer Epidemiology Biomarkers & Prevention*, Vol. 15, 1688-1695, Sept. 2006.

[18] Allain T., et al. Hypovitaminosis D in older adults. *Gerontology*, Vol. 49, No. 5:273-278, Sept-Oct 2003.

[19] Rose, D., et al. Omega-3 fatty acids as cancer chemopreventive agents. *Pharmacology & Therapeutics*, Vol. 83, No. 3:217-244, Sept. 1999.

[20] Hallemeesch, M., et al. Reduced arginine availability and nitric oxide production. Clinical Nutrition, Vol. 21, No. 4:273-279, Aug. 2002.

[21] Burnett, A.L. Role of nitric oxide in the physiology of erection. *Biology of Reproduction*, Vol. 52, No. 3:485-489, March 1995.

[22] Choi, Y.D., et al. The distribution of nitric oxide synthase in human corpus cavernosum on various impotent patients. *Yonsei Medical Journal*, Vol. 38, No. 3:125-132. June 1997.

[23] Huynh, N., et al. Amino Acids, Arginase and Nitric Oxide in Vascular Health. *Clinical and Experimental Pharmacology and Physiology*, Vol. 33, No. 1-2:1, Jan. 2006.

[24] Stuehr, D. Enzymes of the L-Arginine to Nitric Oxide Pathway. *The Journal of Nutrition*, Vol. 134:2748S-2751S, Oct. 2004.

[25] Morris, S. Enzymes of Arginine Metabolism. *The Journal of Nutrition*, Vol. 134:2743S-2747S, Oct. 2004.

[26] Zorgniotti, A.W., et al. Effect of large doses of the nitric oxide precursor, L-arginine, on erectile dysfunction. *International Journal of Impotence Research*, Vol. 6, No.1:33-35. March 1994.

[27] Helzlsouer, K., et al. Association between alpha-tocopherol, gamma-tocopherol, selenium, and subsequent prostate cancer. *Journal of the National Cancer Institute*, Vol. 92, No. 24:2018-2023, Dec. 2000.

[28] Costello, L., et al. Testosterone and prolactin regulation of metabolic genes and citrate metabolism of prostate epithelial cells. *Hormone and Metabolic Research*, Vol. 34, No. 8:417-424, Aug. 2002.

[29] Fortes C., The effect of zinc and vitamin A supplementation on immune response in an older population. *Journal of the American Geriatrics Society*, Vol.46, No. 1:19-26. Jan. 1998.

[30] Shores, M. et al. Low Serum Testosterone and Mortality in Male Veterans. *Archives of Internal Medicine*, Vol. 166, No. 15:1660-1665, Aug 2006.

[31] Morales, A., et al. Endocrine Aspects of Sexual Dysfunction in Men. *The Journal of Sexual Medicine*, Vol. 1, No. 1, July 2004.

[32] Feldman, H.A., et al, Massachusetts Male Aging Study. *Journal of Urology*, Vol. 151, No. 1:54-61, Jan 1994.

[33] Pytel, Y.A., et al. Long-term clinical and biologic effects of the lipidosterolic extract of Serenoa repens in patients with symptomatic benign prostatic hyperplasia. *Advances in Therapy*, Vol. 19, No. 6:297-306. Nov-Dec 2002.

[34] Ishani, A., et al. Pygeum africanum for the treatment of patients with benign prostatic hyperplasia: a systematic review and quantitative meta-analysis. *The American Journal of Medicine*, Vol. 109, No. 8:654-64, Dec. 2000.

[35] Breza, J., et al. Efficacy and acceptability of tadenan (Pygeum africanum extract) in the treatment of benign prostatic hyperplasia (BPH): a multicentre trial in central Europe. *Current Medical Research and Opinion*, Vol. 14, No. 3:127-39, 1998.

[36] Bartlet, A., et al. Efficacy of Pygeum africanum extract in the medical therapy of urination disorders due to benign prostatic hyperplasia: evaluation of objective and subjective parameters. A placebo-controlled double-blind multicenter study. *Wiener klinische Wochenschrift*, Vol. 102, No. 22:667-73. Nov. 1990.

[37] Schleich, S., et al. Activity-Guided Isolation of an Antiandrogenic Compound of Pygeum africanum. *Planta Medica*, Vol. 72:547-551, April 2006.

[38] Wilt, T. Pygeum Africanum for Benign Prostatic Hyperplasia. *Cochrane Review*, July 2006.

[39] Yablonsky, F., et al. Antiproliferative effect of Pygeum africanum extract on rat prostatic fibroblasts. *The Journal of Urology*, Vol. 157, No. 6:2381-2387, June 1997.

[40] Hryb, D.J., et al. The effect of extracts of the roots of the stinging nettle (Urtica dioica) on the interaction of SHBG with its receptor on human prostatic membranes. *Planta Medica*, Vol. 61, No. 1:31-2. Feb. 1995.

[41] Schottner, M., et al. Lignans from the roots of Urtica dioica and their metabolites bind to human sex hormone binding globulin (SHBG). *Planta Medica*, Vol. 63 No. 6:529–532. Dec. 1997.

[42] Dutkiewicz, S. Usefulness of Cernilton in the treatment of benign prostatic hyperplasia. *International Urology and Nephrology*, Vol. 28, No.1:49-53, 1996.

[43] MacDonald, R., et al. A systematic review of Cernilton for the Treatment of benign prostatic hyperplasia. *British Journal of Urology International*, Vol. 85, No. 7:836-841, May 2000.

[44] Wilt, T., et al. Cernilton for benign prostatic hyperplasia. *Cochrane Database of Systematic Reviews*, 2000.

[45] Buck, A.C., et al. Treatment of outflow tract obstruction due to benign prostatic hyperplasia with the pollen extract, cernilton. A double-blind, placebo-controlled study. *British Journal of Urology*, Vol. 66:398-404, 1990.

[46] Yasumoto, R., et al. Clinical evaluation of long-term treatment using cernitin pollen extract in patients with benign prostatic hyperplasia. *Clinical Therapeutics*, Vol. 17, No. 1:82-7 Jan.-Feb. 1995.

[47] Kirby, M., et al. Endothelial dysfunction links erectile dysfunction to heart disease. *International Journal of Clinical Practice*, Vol. 59, No. 2:225-9, Feb. 2005.

[48] Le Bars, P.L., et al. Efficacy and safety of a Ginkgo biloba extract. *Public Health and Nutrition*. Vol. 3 No. 4A:495-499, Dec. 2000.

[49] Salvati, G., et al, Effects of Panax Ginseng saponins on male fertility. *Panminerva Medica*, Vol 38, No. 4:249-254, Dec. 1996.

[50] Choi, Y.D., et al, In vitro and in vivo experimental effect of Korean red ginseng on erection., *Journal of Urology*, Vol. 162, No. 4:1508-1511, Oct. 1999.

[51] Morales, A., et al. Is yohimbine effective in the treatment of organic impotence? Results of a controlled trial., *Journal of Urology*, Vol. 137, No. 6:1168-72, June 1987.

[52] Guay, A., et al, Yohimbine treatment of organic erectile dysfunction in a dose-escalation trial. *International Journal of Impotence Research*, Vol. 14, No. 1:25-31 Feb. 2002.

[53] Pittler, M.H., Yohimbine in therapy of erectile dysfunction., *Fortschritte der Medizin,* Vol. 116, No.1:32-3 Jan.1988

[54] James F. Balch, Phyllis Balch, *Prescription for Nutritional Healing,* 3rd ed., Avery Books, 2000.

[55] Duke, J. *The Green Pharmacy,* St. Martins Press, New York, NY 2001.

[56] Murray, M. and Pizzorno, J. *Encylopedia of Natural Medicine,* 2nd Ed, Prima Publishing, Rocklin, CA 1998.

[57] Betz, J.M., et al. Gas Chromatographic Determination of Yohimbine in Commercial Yohimbe Products. *Journal of the Association of Official Analytical Chemistry International,* Vol. 78, No. 5:1189-1194.

[58] Gonzales, G.F., et al. Effect of Lepidium meyenii (Maca), a root with aphrodisiac and fertility-enhancing properties, on serum reproductive hormone levels in adult healthy men. *The Journal of Endocrinology,* Vol.176, No. 1:163-168, Jan. 2003.

[59] Zheng, B.L., et al. Effect of a lipidic extract from lepidium meyenii on sexual behavior in mice and rats. *Urology,* Vol. 55, No. 4:598-602, April 2000.

[60] Cicero, A.F., et al. Lepidium meyenii Walp. improves sexual behaviour in male rats independently from its action on spontaneous locomotor activity. *Journal of Ethnopharmacology,* Vol. 75, No. 2-3:225-9, May 2001.

[61] Gonzales, G.F., et al. Effect of Lepidium meyenii (maca) roots on spermatogenesis of male rats. *Asian Journal of Andrology,* Vol 3, No. 3:231-233, Sept. 2001.

[62] Kuang, A.K., et al. Effects of yang-restoring herb medicines on the levels of plasma corticosterone, testosterone and triiodothyronine. *Zhong Xi Yi Jie He Za Zhi (Chinese Journal of Modern Developments in Traditional Medicine),* Vol. 9, No. 12:737-8, 710, Dec. 1989.

[63] Tian, L., et al. Effects of icariin on the erectile function and expression of nitrogen oxide synthase isoforms in corpus cavernosum of arterigenic erectile

dysfunction rat model. *Zhonghua yi xue za zhi (Chinese medical journal; Free China ed.)*, Vol. 84, No. 11:954-957, June 2004.

[64] Adimoelja, A., Phytochemicals and the breakthrough of traditional herbs in the management of sexual dysfunctions, *International Journal of Andrology*, Vol. 23, Supp. 2:82-84, 2000.

[65] Adaikan, P.G., et al. Proerectile pharmacological effects of Tribulus terrestris extract on the rabbit corpus cavernosum. *Annals of the Academy of Medicine*, Singapore; 29(1): 22–26, Jan. 2000.

[66] Xu, Y.X., et al. Three new saponins from Tribulus terrestris. *Planta Medica*, Vol. 66, No. 6:545-50, Aug. 2000.

[67] Kostove, I., et al. Two new sulfated furostanol saponins from Tribulus terrestris. *Zeitschrift fur Naturforschung. Journal of biosciences*, Vol. 57, No. 1-2:33-8, Jan.-Feb. 2002.

[68] Lebrett, T., et al. Efficacy and safety of a novel combination of L-arginine glutamate and yohimbine hydrochloride: a new oral therapy for erectile dysfunction. *European Urology*, Vol. 41, No. 6:608-13, June 2002.

[69] Ito, T., et al. The effects of ArginMax, a natural dietary supplement for enhancement of male sexual function. *Hawaii Medical Journal*, Vol. 57, No. 12:741-744, Dec. 1998.

[70] Armanini, D., et al. Reduction of serum testosterone in men by licorice. *New England Journal of Medicine*, Vol. 341, No. 15:1158, Correspondance, Oct. 1999.

[71] Verhamme, K., et al. Nonsteroidal Anti-inflammatory Drugs and Increased Risk of Acute Urinary Retention. *Archives of Internal Medicine*, Vol. 165 No. 13, July 2005.

[72] Chacko, J., et al. Association between marijuana use and transitional cell carcinoma. *Urology*, Vol. 67, No. 1:100-4, Jan. 2006.

[73] Gilad, R., et al. Tonic-clonic seizures in patients taking sildenafil. *British Medical Journal*, Vol. 325, No. 7369:869, Oct. 2002.

[74] Fraunfelder, F, et al, Drug Related Adverse Effects of Clinical Importance to the Opthalmologist. *American Academy of Ophthalmology*, Nov. 2003.

[75] Striano, P., et al. Epileptic seizures can follow high doses of oral vardenafil. *British Medical Journal*, Vol. 333, No. 7574:785, Oct. 2006.

[76] Koussa, S., et al. Epileptic seizures and vardenafil. *Revue Neurologique (Paris)*, Vol. 162, No. 5:651-652, May 2006.

[77] Roizenblatt, S., Et al. A Double-blind, Placebo-Controlled, Crossover Study of Sildenafil in Obstructive Sleep Apnea. *Archives of Internal Medicine*, Vol. 166, No. 16: 1763-1767, Sept. 2006.

[78] Wright, P.J. Comparison of Phosphodiesterase Type 5 (PDE5) Inhibitors. *International Journal of Clinical Practice*, Vol. 60, No. 8:967-975, Aug. 2006.

[79] Ilan Gruenwald, MD, et al, Shockwave Treatment of Erectile Dysfunction, *Therapeutic Advances in Urology*, Vol 5, No. 2:95-99, 2013

[80] Gruenwald I, et al, Low-intensity extracorporeal shock wave therapy—a novel effective treatment for erectile dysfunction in severe ED patients who respond poorly to PDE5 inhibitor therapy, *Journal of Sexual Medicine*, Vol 9, No 1:259-64, Jan 2012

[81] Noam. D. Kitry, et al, Low Intensity Shock Wave Treatment for Erectile Dysfunction—How Long Does the Effect Last?, *American Urolological Association, Journal of Urology, Volume 200, Issue 1, Pages 167–170, July 2018*

[82] Yoram Vardi, Et al, Can Low-Intensity Extracorporeal Shockwave Therapy Improve Erectile Function? A 6-Month Follow-up Pilot Study in Patients with Organic Erectile Dysfunction, *European Eurology*, Vol 58:243-248, April 2010

[83] Drogo K Montague, MD, Penile Prosthesis Implantation for End-Stage Erectile Dysfunction after Radical Prostatectomy, *Reviews in Urology*, Vol 7, No. 2:S51–S57, 2005.

Don't miss out!

Visit the website below and you can sign up to receive emails whenever James Occhiogrosso publishes a new book. There's no charge and no obligation.

https://books2read.com/r/B-A-AOZG-UIFV

BOOKS 2 READ

Connecting independent readers to independent writers.

Also by James Occhiogrosso

Solutions for Erectile Dysfunction
Your Prostate, Your Libido, Your Life

Watch for more at www.prostatehealthnaturally.com/index.html.

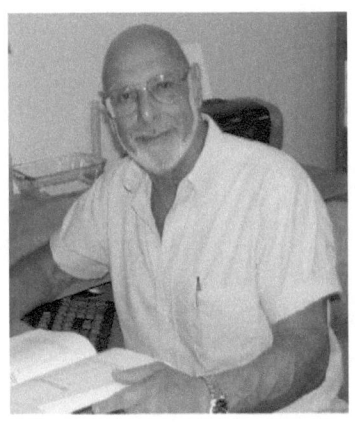

About the Author

Author bio: James Occhiogrosso, N.D. is a Natural Health Practitioner specializing in male and female health issues and author of the book "Your Prostate, Your Libido, Your Life" and others. He maintains an active practice helping both men and women overcome hormonal and sexual issues associated with aging, including loss of libido, erectile dysfunction and menopausal problems, and often acts as an advisor for men with prostate cancer whose doctors recommend a "watchful waiting" approach. Salivary home hormone test kits as well as bio-identical hormone creams are available at his website.

He lives with his wife of nearly 40 years in Southwest Florida, USA.

Connect with him at: DrJim@HealthNaturallyToday.com

Cover photo by ?? ??

Read more at www.prostatehealthnaturally.com/index.html.

www.ingramcontent.com/pod-product-compliance
Lightning Source LLC
Chambersburg PA
CBHW020327290526
45785CB00007B/2949

* 9 7 8 1 3 8 6 3 4 6 9 9 9 *